FU to Getting Old: A Guide to Staying Youthful After 40

I. Introduction

A. Embracing a positive mindset towards aging

Embracing a positive mindset towards aging is crucial for staying young at heart. Here are some key points to consider:

1. Acceptance: Recognize that aging is a natural part of life and that everyone goes through it. Embrace the changes that come with age, both physically and mentally.

2. Gratitude: Focus on the positive aspects of getting older and appreciate the experiences and wisdom gained over the years. Cultivate a sense of gratitude for the opportunities and achievements that have come your way.

3. Self-care: Prioritize self-care in your daily routine. Take care of your physical, emotional, and mental well-being. Engage in activities that bring you joy and help you relax, such as hobbies, meditation, or spending time in nature.

4. Positive self-talk: Be mindful of your inner dialogue and challenge negative thoughts about aging. Replace self-limiting beliefs with uplifting and empowering affirmations that reinforce your worth, capabilities, and potential.

5. Surround yourself with positivity: Surround yourself with people who uplift and inspire you. Seek out social connections that bring joy, support, and encouragement. Engage in activities that foster a positive and vibrant community.

6. Stay active: Engaging in regular physical activity not only benefits your physical health but also boosts your mood and mental well-being. Find activities you enjoy and make them a part of your

routine. It could be walking, dancing, yoga, or any form of exercise that brings you pleasure.

7. Embrace new challenges: Keep learning and trying new things. Engaging in new experiences stimulates the brain and keeps you mentally sharp. Whether it's learning a new language, taking up a new hobby, or traveling to new places, embracing new challenges keeps life exciting and keeps you feeling youthful.

Remember, your mindset plays a significant role in how you experience the aging process. By embracing a positive mindset, you can maintain a youthful spirit and approach life with enthusiasm and vitality.

B. Importance of staying active and feeling young

Staying active and feeling young go hand in hand, as they both contribute to a fulfilling and vibrant life. Here are some reasons why staying active is important for maintaining a youthful mindset:

1. Physical health: Regular physical activity helps improve cardiovascular health, strengthen muscles and bones, and maintain a healthy weight. It boosts energy levels, increases mobility, and reduces the risk of chronic illnesses such as heart disease, diabetes, and certain cancers.

2. Mental well-being: Physical activity releases endorphins, which are known as "feel-good" hormones. Regular exercise helps reduce stress, anxiety, and symptoms of depression. It improves cognitive function, memory, and overall brain health, keeping your mind sharp and focused.

3. Increased vitality: Staying active helps improve stamina and endurance, allowing you to engage in daily activities with ease. It enhances balance, coordination, and flexibility, reducing the risk of falls and injuries. By maintaining physical vitality, you can continue to pursue your passions and enjoy an active lifestyle.

4. Social connections: Participating in physical activities often provides opportunities for social interactions. Whether it's joining a

sports team, attending fitness classes, or going for group walks, staying active can help you meet new people, build friendships, and strengthen existing relationships. Social connections contribute to a sense of belonging and overall well-being.

5. Positive mindset: Engaging in regular exercise and physical activity helps release stress, boosts mood, and promotes a positive outlook. It can increase self-confidence, improve body image, and enhance self-esteem. Feeling good about yourself and your physical abilities can contribute to a more youthful and positive mindset.

6. Longevity: Research consistently shows that staying active is associated with a longer and healthier life. Regular exercise and physical activity can help prevent age-related decline, improve quality of life, and increase life expectancy. By maintaining an active lifestyle, you have a better chance of enjoying your later years with vitality and independence.

Remember, staying active doesn't necessarily mean intense workouts or pushing yourself beyond your limits. Find activities that you enjoy and that suit your fitness level. Whether it's walking, swimming, dancing, gardening, or any other form of movement, the key is to find something that keeps you engaged and motivated. By staying active, you can continue to feel young, vibrant, and full of life.

II. Mindset Shift

A. Changing the perception of age as a limitation

Changing the perception of age as a limitation is crucial for promoting a more inclusive and positive society. Here are some ways we can challenge age-related stereotypes and embrace the idea that age is not a barrier:

1. Celebrate diverse experiences: Each stage of life brings unique experiences and wisdom. By recognizing and valuing the contributions of people of all ages, we can foster a culture that respects and appreciates the richness that comes with different life

stages. This includes giving older adults opportunities to share their knowledge and skills with younger generations.

2. Promote lifelong learning: Encouraging continuous learning and personal growth at every age is essential. Emphasize the importance of intellectual curiosity and provide access to educational resources and opportunities for people of all ages. This can include workshops, classes, online courses, and mentorship programs that facilitate intergenerational learning.

3. Challenge ageist language and attitudes: Language plays a significant role in shaping our perceptions. Avoid using derogatory terms or age-related stereotypes when referring to older adults. Instead, use respectful and inclusive language that highlights the individuality and capabilities of people regardless of their age.

4. Embrace intergenerational connections: Encouraging interactions between different age groups can break down barriers and foster understanding. Promote activities that bring people of different ages together, such as community projects, volunteering opportunities, or mentorship programs. By fostering intergenerational connections, we can learn from one another and build empathy and respect.

5. Highlight positive examples: Share stories and examples of individuals who have defied age-related stereotypes and achieved remarkable things. Highlighting these positive role models can inspire others and challenge the notion that age limits our potential. By showcasing older adults who are thriving in various fields and pursuits, we can shift the narrative around aging.

6. Advocate for age-inclusive policies: Encourage policymakers to implement age-inclusive policies that promote equal opportunities and access to resources for people of all ages. This can include healthcare policies, employment practices, and social support systems that recognize and address the diverse needs and capabilities of individuals across the lifespan.

Changing the perception of age as a limitation requires a collective effort from individuals, communities, and institutions. By challenging stereotypes, promoting inclusivity, and celebrating the contributions of people of all ages, we can create a society that values and embraces individuals at every stage of life.

B. Cultivating a positive attitude towards aging

Cultivating a positive attitude towards aging is important for our overall well-being and can greatly enhance our quality of life as we grow older. Here are some tips to help foster a positive outlook on aging:

1. Embrace self-care: Taking care of ourselves physically, mentally, and emotionally is essential at any age. Prioritize activities that promote well-being, such as regular exercise, nutritious eating, getting enough rest, and engaging in activities that bring joy and fulfillment.

2. Focus on the positives: Instead of dwelling on the limitations that may come with aging, shift your mindset towards the positives. Recognize and appreciate the wisdom, experience, and resilience that often accompany getting older. Celebrate the milestones and achievements you've reached throughout your life.

3. Stay socially connected: Maintaining strong social connections is crucial for a positive aging experience. Nurture relationships with family, friends, and your community. Seek out opportunities to connect with others, whether through joining clubs or organizations, volunteering, or participating in social activities. Engaging with others can help combat feelings of isolation and contribute to a sense of purpose and belonging.

4. Set new goals and pursue passions: Aging doesn't mean giving up on dreams or aspirations. Set new goals and pursue activities that bring you joy and fulfillment. Whether it's learning a new skill, exploring a hobby, or embarking on a new adventure, having goals and passions to pursue can keep you engaged and excited about life.

5. Challenge age-related stereotypes: Don't let societal expectations or stereotypes define what aging means for you. Challenge negative assumptions and beliefs about aging by actively engaging in

activities that defy those stereotypes. Lead by example and show others that age is not a barrier to living a fulfilling and meaningful life.

6. Seek support when needed: It's important to recognize that aging can come with unique challenges, and it's okay to ask for help or seek support when needed. Whether it's addressing health concerns, seeking advice on financial matters, or accessing community resources, reaching out for support can make a significant difference in your overall well-being.

Remember, cultivating a positive attitude towards aging is a mindset that can be nurtured and developed. By focusing on self-care, staying socially connected, pursuing passions, challenging stereotypes, and seeking support when needed, you can embrace aging with optimism and enjoy a fulfilling and meaningful life at any age.

C. Setting new goals and embracing new opportunities

Setting new goals and embracing new opportunities is a wonderful way to keep growing and evolving throughout your life. Here are some tips to help you in this process:

1. Reflect on your passions and interests: Take some time to think about the things that truly excite and inspire you. What are your passions and interests? What activities or hobbies bring you joy? Identifying these areas will help you set meaningful goals that align with your values and desires.

2. Set SMART goals: SMART stands for Specific, Measurable, Achievable, Relevant, and Time-bound. When setting goals, make sure they are specific and clearly defined. Break them down into smaller, measurable steps that are achievable within a reasonable timeframe. Ensure that your goals are relevant to your interests and aspirations.

3. Step out of your comfort zone: Embracing new opportunities often requires stepping out of your comfort zone. Don't be afraid to try new things or take on challenges. Pushing yourself beyond what

feels familiar can lead to personal growth and open doors to exciting experiences and achievements.

4. Seek inspiration and learning: Surround yourself with sources of inspiration and learning. Read books, listen to podcasts, attend workshops or classes, and engage with people who inspire you. Continuous learning and exposure to new ideas can spark creativity and help you discover new passions and opportunities.

5. Stay adaptable and open-minded: Life is full of unexpected twists and turns. Embrace a mindset of adaptability and open-mindedness to make the most of new opportunities as they arise. Be willing to adjust your goals and plans if needed, and view challenges as opportunities for growth and learning.

6. Celebrate progress and small victories: Acknowledge and celebrate your progress along the way. Every step forward, no matter how small, is a victory. Recognize and appreciate the effort and dedication you put into pursuing your goals and embracing new opportunities.

7. Seek support and collaboration: Don't hesitate to seek support from others. Surround yourself with a supportive network of family, friends, mentors, or like-minded individuals who can offer guidance, encouragement, and accountability. Collaboration and shared experiences can enhance the journey of setting and achieving goals.

Remember, setting new goals and embracing new opportunities is a lifelong process. Be patient with yourself, stay curious, and embrace the journey of personal growth and self-discovery. By stepping outside your comfort zone and pursuing your passions, you can create a fulfilling and vibrant life filled with new experiences and achievements.

III. Exercise for Overall Health

A. Importance of regular physical activity

Regular physical activity is of utmost importance for maintaining a healthy and balanced lifestyle. Here are some key reasons why incorporating regular physical activity into your routine is beneficial:

1. Physical health: Engaging in regular physical activity has numerous health benefits. It helps to reduce the risk of chronic diseases such as heart disease, high blood pressure, type 2 diabetes, and certain types of cancer. Regular exercise also improves cardiovascular health, strengthens muscles and bones, and enhances overall physical fitness.

2. Mental well-being: Physical activity is not only good for the body but also for the mind. Exercise releases endorphins, which are known as "feel-good" hormones, promoting a positive mood and reducing feelings of stress, anxiety, and depression. Regular physical activity can boost self-esteem, improve cognitive function, and enhance sleep quality, leading to overall better mental well-being.

3. Weight management: Engaging in regular physical activity helps in achieving and maintaining a healthy weight. Physical activity helps to burn calories, increase metabolism, and build lean muscle mass. It also contributes to better body composition by reducing body fat and increasing muscle tone, leading to improved body shape and increased energy levels.

4. Increased energy levels: Contrary to what one might think, regular physical activity actually increases energy levels rather than depleting them. Exercise improves blood circulation, enhances oxygen and nutrient delivery to the muscles and tissues, and improves overall energy production within the body. As a result, individuals who are physically active often experience increased stamina and vitality in their daily lives.

5. Improved brain function: Physical activity has a positive impact on brain health and cognitive function. Exercise promotes the growth of new brain cells, improves memory, attention, and concentration, and enhances overall cognitive performance. Regular physical activity has also been linked to a reduced risk of age-related

cognitive decline and neurodegenerative diseases such as Alzheimer's.

6. Social benefits: Participating in physical activities often involves social interaction, whether it's joining a sports team, attending group fitness classes, or simply going for a walk with friends or family. Engaging in physical activity with others can foster social connections, improve social skills, and create a sense of belonging and community.

7. Longevity and quality of life: Regular physical activity is associated with a longer and healthier life. Studies have shown that individuals who are physically active have a lower risk of premature death and a higher likelihood of maintaining independence and functional abilities as they age. Regular exercise contributes to an overall improved quality of life by enhancing physical, mental, and emotional well-being.

Incorporating regular physical activity into your daily routine doesn't have to be complicated or time-consuming. Even small changes such as taking the stairs instead of the elevator, going for a brisk walk during lunch breaks, or participating in enjoyable activities like dancing or gardening can make a significant difference. Remember, every bit of physical activity counts, and the benefits are well worth the effort.

B. Choosing activities that suit personal preferences and abilities

When it comes to choosing physical activities, it's important to consider your personal preferences and abilities. Here are some factors to keep in mind:

1. Interests and enjoyment: Select activities that you genuinely enjoy and find interesting. Whether it's dancing, swimming, hiking, playing a sport, or practicing yoga, engaging in activities that you like will increase your motivation and make it more likely for you to stick with them in the long run.

2. Fitness level and abilities: Consider your current fitness level and physical abilities. Choose activities that are appropriate for your age, fitness level, and any existing health conditions. If you're a beginner, start with low-impact activities and gradually increase the intensity and duration as your fitness improves.

3. Variety and balance: Incorporate a variety of activities to keep things interesting and to engage different muscle groups. This can help prevent boredom and reduce the risk of overuse injuries. Additionally, aim for a balance between cardiovascular exercises (such as brisk walking, running, or cycling) and strength-training exercises (such as weightlifting, resistance training, or bodyweight exercises) to promote overall fitness and muscle strength.

4. Accessibility and convenience: Consider the accessibility and convenience of the activities you choose. Opt for activities that fit easily into your daily routine and can be done in your local area or at home. This can help overcome barriers and make it more likely for you to consistently engage in physical activity.

5. Social opportunities: Some activities provide opportunities for social interaction, which can enhance motivation and enjoyment. Joining a sports team, attending group fitness classes, or participating in recreational activities with friends or family can make exercise more enjoyable and provide a sense of social connection.

6. Safety considerations: Prioritize activities that are safe and suitable for your physical condition. If you have any health concerns or limitations, consult with a healthcare professional or a qualified exercise specialist to ensure that you choose activities that are appropriate and safe for you.

Remember, the goal is to find activities that you genuinely enjoy and can incorporate into your lifestyle. Experiment with different activities, be open to trying new things, and listen to your body to find the right balance between challenge and enjoyment. Regular physical activity should be a sustainable and enjoyable part of your life, supporting your overall health and well-being.

C. Incorporating cardio, strength training, and flexibility exercises

Incorporating a mix of cardio, strength training, and flexibility exercises into your fitness routine is a great way to achieve overall fitness and improve your health. Here are some tips to help you include these different types of exercises:

1. Cardiovascular exercises: Cardio exercises raise your heart rate and increase your breathing, helping to improve your cardiovascular health and burn calories. Some examples include brisk walking, running, cycling, swimming, dancing, or aerobics. Aim for at least 150 minutes of moderate-intensity cardio exercise or 75 minutes of vigorous-intensity cardio exercise per week. You can break it down into smaller sessions throughout the week if needed.

2. Strength training exercises: Strength training helps build and tone muscles, increases bone density, and boosts metabolism. It involves using resistance to challenge your muscles. You can use free weights, weight machines, resistance bands, or even your body weight. Aim to include strength training exercises for all major muscle groups at least twice a week. This can include exercises like squats, lunges, push-ups, pull-ups, or using weights for bicep curls or shoulder presses.

3. Flexibility exercises: Flexibility exercises help improve your range of motion, prevent injuries, and promote better posture. Examples include stretching exercises, yoga, Pilates, or tai chi. Make sure to incorporate stretches for all major muscle groups in your body, holding each stretch for 15-30 seconds without bouncing. It's best to do flexibility exercises at least two to three times per week.

4. Balancing your routine: Aim to have a well-rounded routine that includes all three types of exercises. You can alternate between cardio and strength training on different days or even combine them in circuit-style workouts. It's also important to include flexibility exercises either as part of your warm-up or cool-down routine.

5. Progression and variety: As you become more comfortable with your routine, gradually increase the intensity, duration, or resistance of your exercises to continue challenging yourself. Additionally, try to vary your exercises to prevent boredom and to engage different muscle groups.

6. Listen to your body: Pay attention to how your body feels during and after exercise. If you experience pain or discomfort, modify or stop the exercise and seek guidance from a healthcare professional or a qualified trainer. It's important to exercise safely and within your abilities.

Remember, consistency is key. Aim for a minimum of 150 minutes of moderate-intensity cardio, two strength training sessions, and regular flexibility exercises each week. Adjust the frequency, duration, and intensity of your workouts based on your goals, preferences, and fitness level. Stay motivated by finding activities you enjoy and gradually challenging yourself to reach new milestones.

IV. Cardiovascular Fitness

A. Benefits of cardiovascular exercise for heart health

Cardiovascular exercise, also known as aerobic exercise, offers numerous benefits for heart health. Here are some of the key benefits:

1. Strengthening the heart: Cardio exercises, such as brisk walking, running, cycling, or swimming, increase your heart rate and make it work harder. Over time, this strengthens the heart muscle, making it more efficient at pumping blood throughout the body.

2. Improving heart health: Regular cardio exercise can help reduce the risk of heart disease by lowering blood pressure and cholesterol levels. It also promotes healthy blood flow, reduces inflammation, and improves the function of blood vessels.

3. Increasing oxygen supply: Cardio activities increase the demand for oxygen in your body. Through regular aerobic exercise, your

body becomes more efficient at using oxygen, which helps deliver oxygen-rich blood to the muscles and organs, including the heart.

4. Managing weight: Cardio exercise is an effective way to burn calories and maintain a healthy weight. Excess weight puts strain on the heart and increases the risk of heart disease. Engaging in regular cardio workouts can help control weight and reduce the risk of obesity-related heart problems.

5. Enhancing circulation: Cardio exercises stimulate blood circulation, improving the flow of oxygen and nutrients to the body's tissues. This can help prevent the buildup of plaque in the arteries, reducing the risk of conditions like atherosclerosis and heart attacks.

6. Reducing stress and improving mental health: Cardiovascular exercise releases endorphins, the "feel-good" hormones, which can help reduce stress, anxiety, and symptoms of depression. Improved mental well-being is closely linked to heart health.

7. Boosting energy levels: Regular cardio workouts increase stamina and endurance, allowing you to perform daily activities with less fatigue. This energy boost can enhance overall quality of life and make physical tasks easier to accomplish.

Remember, it's important to consult with a healthcare professional before starting any new exercise program, especially if you have any underlying health conditions. They can provide personalized advice and guidance based on your specific needs and limitations.

B. Suitable activities for individuals over 40 (e.g., walking, swimming, cycling)

There are many suitable activities for individuals over 40 that offer health benefits and are generally low-impact. Here are a few examples:

1. Walking: Walking is a simple and accessible exercise that can be done almost anywhere. It is gentle on the joints, helps improve cardiovascular health, and can be easily incorporated into your daily routine.

2. Swimming: Swimming is a low-impact, full-body workout that is easy on the joints. It provides cardiovascular benefits, strengthens muscles, and improves flexibility. It is particularly beneficial for individuals with joint pain or arthritis.

3. Cycling: Cycling is a great cardiovascular exercise that is gentle on the joints and offers a variety of options. You can cycle outdoors, join a cycling group, or use a stationary bike at home or in a gym. It helps improve leg strength, endurance, and overall fitness.

4. Yoga or Pilates: These activities focus on flexibility, balance, and core strength. They can help improve posture, reduce muscle stiffness, and enhance overall body awareness. Yoga and Pilates classes specifically designed for individuals over 40 are available and can be beneficial.

5. Strength training: Engaging in regular strength training exercises, such as lifting weights or using resistance bands, helps maintain muscle mass, increase bone density, and improve metabolism. It can also help prevent age-related muscle loss and maintain overall strength and functionality.

6. Dancing: Dancing is a fun and enjoyable way to stay active. It improves cardiovascular health, coordination, and balance. There are various dance styles to choose from, such as Zumba, salsa, or ballroom dancing.

7. Tai Chi: Tai Chi is a gentle martial art that incorporates slow, flowing movements, deep breathing, and meditation. It helps improve balance, flexibility, and relaxation. Tai Chi is suitable for people of all fitness levels and can be particularly beneficial for older adults.

Remember to listen to your body and choose activities that you enjoy and that align with your fitness level and any specific health considerations. It's always a good idea to consult with a healthcare professional or a certified fitness instructor to ensure you are engaging in activities that are safe and appropriate for you.

C. Setting goals and gradually increasing intensity

Setting goals and gradually increasing intensity is a smart approach to ensure progress and avoid injury when engaging in physical activities. Here's how you can do it:

1. Define your goals: Determine what you want to achieve through your physical activities. It could be improving cardiovascular fitness, increasing strength, losing weight, or simply feeling more energized. Make your goals specific, measurable, attainable, relevant, and time-bound (SMART).

2. Start small: Begin with activities that are comfortable for your current fitness level. For example, if you're walking, start with shorter distances or durations and gradually increase them over time. This allows your body to adapt and reduces the risk of overexertion.

3. Gradually increase intensity: Once you've established a baseline, progressively challenge yourself by increasing the intensity, duration, or frequency of your activities. For instance, you can increase your walking pace, add intervals of higher intensity, or extend your workout time. Gradual increments help your body adapt and build strength and endurance.

4. Listen to your body: Pay attention to how your body feels during and after physical activities. If you experience pain, excessive fatigue, or discomfort, it may indicate that you're pushing yourself too hard. Adjust the intensity or duration accordingly, and consult a healthcare professional if necessary.

5. Set milestones: Break your long-term goals into smaller milestones. Celebrate each milestone achieved, as it will help keep you motivated and engaged. For example, if your goal is to run a 5K, set smaller milestones like running for 10 minutes without stopping, increasing your distance gradually, and finally completing the 5K.

6. Track your progress: Keep a record of your activities, noting the duration, intensity, and any milestones reached. This allows you to see your progress over time and identify areas where you can push yourself further.

7. Adjust as needed: As you progress, you may need to adjust your goals and intensity levels. Be flexible and adapt your plan to suit your changing needs and circumstances.

Remember, it's important to listen to your body, take rest days when needed, and seek guidance from professionals if you have any specific health concerns or conditions. By setting realistic goals and gradually increasing intensity, you can make consistent progress and enjoy the benefits of an active lifestyle.

V. Strength Training

A. Importance of maintaining muscle mass and strength

Maintaining muscle mass and strength is crucial for overall health and well-being. Here are some key reasons why it's important:

1. Functional independence: Strong muscles allow you to perform daily activities with ease, such as carrying groceries, climbing stairs, or getting up from a chair. Maintaining muscle mass and strength helps you maintain functional independence as you age, reducing the risk of falls and improving your overall quality of life.

2. Metabolism and weight management: Muscle is more metabolically active than fat, meaning it burns more calories at rest. By maintaining muscle mass, you can support a healthy metabolism and make it easier to manage your weight. This is especially important as we age since we tend to naturally lose muscle mass, leading to a slower metabolism.

3. Bone health: Strength training and maintaining muscle mass help support bone health. Resistance exercises put stress on the bones, stimulating them to become stronger. This can help prevent or manage conditions like osteoporosis and reduce the risk of fractures.

4. Injury prevention: Strong muscles act as protective support for your joints and ligaments, reducing the risk of injuries. They help stabilize your body during movements, improving balance and coordination. This is particularly important for athletes or individuals participating in physical activities.

5. Chronic disease management: Regular resistance training, which helps maintain muscle mass and strength, has been associated with improved management of chronic conditions such as diabetes, heart disease, and arthritis. It can help control blood sugar levels, lower blood pressure, improve cholesterol profiles, and reduce joint pain.

6. Mental well-being: Engaging in strength training and maintaining muscle mass has positive effects on mental health. Physical activity releases endorphins, which can boost mood and reduce symptoms of anxiety and depression. Additionally, feeling physically strong and capable can improve self-confidence and overall self-esteem.

7. Aging gracefully: As mentioned earlier, muscle loss is a natural part of the aging process. However, by maintaining muscle mass and strength through regular exercise, you can slow down this decline and age more gracefully. It can help preserve muscle tone, posture, and overall physical function, allowing you to maintain an active and independent lifestyle.

Overall, maintaining muscle mass and strength is essential for various aspects of health and well-being. Incorporating regular resistance training, along with a balanced diet, can help you achieve and maintain optimal muscle health throughout your life.

B. Different types of strength training exercises (e.g., weightlifting, resistance bands, bodyweight exercises)

There are several types of strength training exercises that you can incorporate into your fitness routine. Here are a few examples:

1. Weightlifting: Weightlifting typically involves using barbells, dumbbells, or kettlebells to perform exercises that target specific muscle groups. This can include exercises like squats, deadlifts, bench presses, and shoulder presses. Weightlifting allows you to progressively increase the load, challenging your muscles and promoting strength gains.

2. Resistance bands: Resistance bands are elastic bands that provide resistance when stretched. They come in different levels of resistance, allowing you to adjust the intensity of your workout.

Resistance bands can be used for a wide range of exercises, including bicep curls, tricep extensions, lateral band walks, and glute bridges. They are portable, versatile, and can be used for both upper and lower body workouts.

3. Bodyweight exercises: Bodyweight exercises use your own body weight as resistance. These exercises can be done anywhere and require no equipment. Examples of bodyweight exercises include push-ups, squats, lunges, planks, burpees, and mountain climbers. Bodyweight exercises can effectively target multiple muscle groups and improve overall strength and stability.

4. Suspension training: Suspension training involves using suspension straps, such as TRX, to perform exercises that leverage your body weight and gravity. These exercises engage multiple muscle groups simultaneously and challenge your core stability. Suspension training exercises can include rows, chest presses, squats, lunges, and planks.

5. Plyometric exercises: Plyometric exercises are explosive movements that involve quick, powerful muscle contractions. They help improve power and athletic performance. Examples include box jumps, jump squats, burpees, and medicine ball throws. Plyometric exercises can be intense, so it's important to have a solid foundation of strength and proper form before incorporating them into your routine.

6. Isometric exercises: Isometric exercises involve static muscle contractions without any joint movement. These exercises help improve muscular endurance and stability. Examples include planks, wall sits, and glute bridges. Isometric exercises can be done with or without equipment and are beneficial for strengthening the core and postural muscles.

Remember, it's important to choose exercises that are appropriate for your fitness level and goals. Consult with a fitness professional or trainer if you're unsure about proper form or if you have any specific concerns or limitations. They can help design a strength training program tailored to your needs.

C. Recommendations for frequency and intensity

When it comes to strength training, finding the right frequency and intensity that works for you is important for achieving your fitness goals while also allowing for proper recovery. Here are some recommendations:

1. Frequency: Aim to incorporate strength training exercises into your routine at least two to three times per week. This frequency allows for enough stimulus to promote strength gains while giving your muscles time to recover between sessions. You can alternate muscle groups on different days or follow a full-body workout routine, depending on your preference and time availability.

2. Intensity: The intensity of your strength training exercises refers to the level of effort or resistance you use. It's important to challenge your muscles to promote strength gains, but also to avoid overexertion or injury. Here are a few ways to adjust the intensity:

- Weight selection: When weightlifting, choose a weight that is challenging enough to complete the desired number of repetitions with good form, but not so heavy that you sacrifice proper technique. Gradually increase the weight as you get stronger.

- Resistance level: With resistance bands or suspension training, choose a band or strap that provides enough resistance to make the exercises challenging, but still allows you to maintain proper form throughout the movement. You can use bands with different levels of resistance to adjust the intensity.

- Progression: As you get stronger, gradually increase the difficulty of your exercises by adding more weight, using more challenging variations, or increasing the number of repetitions or sets. This progressive overload helps to continually challenge your muscles and promote strength gains.

Remember to listen to your body and avoid pushing yourself too hard. Allow for adequate rest and recovery between sessions, especially if you're new to strength training or if you're experiencing muscle soreness. If you're unsure about the appropriate intensity or frequency for your individual needs, consider consulting with a fitness professional who can provide personalized guidance based on your goals, fitness level, and any specific considerations you may have.

VI. Flexibility and Balance

A. Maintaining joint mobility and preventing injuries

Maintaining joint mobility and preventing injuries are vital aspects of any fitness routine. Here are some recommendations to help you achieve these goals:

1. Warm-up: Always start your workouts with a proper warm-up. This can include light cardio exercises like jogging or cycling to increase blood flow and raise your body temperature. Additionally, incorporating dynamic stretches that target the muscles and joints you'll be using during your workout can help prepare your body for the upcoming movements.

2. Stretching: Include both dynamic and static stretches in your routine. Dynamic stretches involve controlled movements that mimic the exercises you'll be performing, helping to increase joint mobility and prepare your muscles for activity. Static stretches should be done after your workout when your muscles are warm. Focus on stretching the major muscle groups and hold each stretch for 15-30 seconds without bouncing.

3. Proper form and technique: When performing exercises, pay close attention to your form and technique. Proper alignment and execution of movements can help reduce the risk of joint injuries. If you're unsure about the correct form, consider working with a qualified fitness professional who can guide and correct your technique.

4. Gradual progression: Avoid jumping into high-intensity workouts or lifting heavy weights without gradually building up your strength and endurance. Gradually increase the intensity, duration, and

weight of your exercises to allow your body to adapt and minimize the risk of overloading your joints.

5. Cross-training and variety: Incorporate a variety of exercises into your routine to avoid overuse injuries. Cross-training helps to improve overall fitness and balance the stress placed on your joints. Include activities like swimming, cycling, or yoga to work different muscle groups and reduce the impact on specific joints.

6. Listen to your body: Pay attention to any pain or discomfort during exercise. If you experience sharp or persistent pain, stop the activity and consult with a healthcare professional. Pushing through pain can lead to further injury and setbacks.

7. Recovery and rest: Allow your body sufficient time to recover and rest between workouts. Adequate rest is essential for joint health and overall recovery. Incorporate regular rest days into your routine and prioritize sleep to support your body's healing and regeneration processes.

Remember, if you have any existing joint conditions or concerns, it's always a good idea to consult with a healthcare professional or physical therapist who can provide personalized advice and modifications tailored to your specific needs.

B. Incorporating activities like yoga, Pilates, or tai chi

Incorporating activities like yoga, Pilates, or tai chi into your fitness routine can be highly beneficial for maintaining joint mobility and preventing injuries. Here's why:

1. Yoga: Yoga focuses on flexibility, balance, and strength, making it an excellent choice for improving joint mobility. The various poses and movements in yoga help to stretch and strengthen the muscles surrounding the joints, promoting flexibility and reducing stiffness. Additionally, yoga emphasizes body awareness and proper alignment, which can help prevent injuries by ensuring correct form and reducing unnecessary strain on the joints.

2. Pilates: Pilates is a low-impact exercise method that targets the core muscles, including those surrounding the spine, hips, and shoulders. By strengthening these muscles, Pilates helps improve stability and alignment, which can reduce the risk of joint injuries. The controlled and precise movements in Pilates also promote body awareness and proper alignment, enhancing joint mobility and reducing the likelihood of overuse injuries.

3. Tai Chi: Tai chi is a gentle and flowing martial art that focuses on slow, deliberate movements and deep breathing. It promotes balance, flexibility, and relaxation, making it suitable for people of all fitness levels. Tai chi's gentle nature is particularly beneficial for individuals with joint issues, as it helps improve range of motion, joint stability, and overall body awareness. Additionally, tai chi's emphasis on slow, controlled movements can reduce the risk of joint strain or sudden impact injuries.

Incorporating these activities into your fitness routine can offer numerous benefits for joint health. However, it's important to start at an appropriate level and progress gradually to avoid overexertion or injury. If you're new to these activities, consider taking classes or working with a qualified instructor who can guide you through proper techniques and modifications based on your individual needs and abilities.

C. Stretching exercises for flexibility and balance improvement

Stretching exercises can be highly effective for improving flexibility and balance. Here are a few examples to incorporate into your routine:

1. Hamstring Stretch: Sit on the floor with one leg extended in front of you and the other leg bent with the sole of your foot against the inner thigh of the extended leg. Lean forward from your hips, reaching for your toes while keeping your back straight. Hold the stretch for 20-30 seconds and repeat on the other side. This stretch targets the hamstrings, which can improve flexibility in the back of your legs.

2. Quadriceps Stretch: Stand upright and hold onto a stable surface for support if needed. Bend one knee and bring your heel towards your buttocks, grasping your ankle or foot with your hand. Keep your standing leg slightly bent and your knees close together. Hold the stretch for 20-30 seconds and repeat on the other side. This stretch targets the quadriceps muscles, promoting flexibility in the front of your thighs.

3. Calf Stretch: Stand facing a wall or sturdy object, placing both hands against it at shoulder height. Extend one leg behind you, keeping the heel on the ground and the knee straight. Lean forward, pressing your hips toward the wall until you feel a stretch in your calf. Hold the stretch for 20-30 seconds and repeat on the other side. This stretch targets the calf muscles, which can improve ankle flexibility and balance.

4. Standing Side Stretch: Stand with your feet hip-width apart and raise both arms overhead. Interlace your fingers and invert your palms, stretching upward. Keeping your feet planted, gently lean to one side, lengthening the opposite side of your body. Hold the stretch for 20-30 seconds and repeat on the other side. This stretch targets the sides of your torso, promoting flexibility and balance.

Remember to warm up your body before stretching and never push yourself to the point of pain. Aim to stretch regularly, ideally after a workout or when your muscles are warmed up. If you're new to stretching or have any specific concerns, it's always a good idea to consult with a fitness professional or physical therapist who can provide guidance and ensure proper technique.

VII. Nutrition and Hydration

A. Importance of a balanced diet for overall health

Maintaining a balanced diet is crucial for achieving and maintaining overall health. Here are some key reasons why a balanced diet is important:

1. Nutrient Intake: A balanced diet ensures that your body receives all the essential nutrients it needs to function optimally. This includes carbohydrates, proteins, healthy fats, vitamins, minerals, and fiber. Each nutrient plays a vital role in supporting various bodily functions, such as energy production, immunity, growth, repair, and regulation of bodily processes.

2. Energy and Performance: Eating a balanced diet provides you with the energy required for daily activities and optimal physical and mental performance. Carbohydrates are the primary source of energy, while proteins and fats provide sustained energy and support muscle function. A well-balanced diet helps maintain stable blood sugar levels, preventing energy crashes and promoting focus and productivity.

3. Disease Prevention: A balanced diet rich in fruits, vegetables, whole grains, lean proteins, and healthy fats is associated with a lower risk of chronic diseases, including heart disease, diabetes, obesity, and certain types of cancer. Nutrient-dense foods provide antioxidants, phytochemicals, and other compounds that help protect against cellular damage, inflammation, and oxidative stress.

4. Weight Management: A balanced diet is essential for achieving and maintaining a healthy weight. It promotes portion control, provides satiety, and prevents excessive calorie consumption. By including a variety of nutrient-dense foods and minimizing processed and high-calorie foods, a balanced diet supports weight loss or weight maintenance goals.

5. Digestive Health: A balanced diet that includes adequate fiber helps maintain a healthy digestive system. Fiber adds bulk to the diet, prevents constipation, and supports regular bowel movements. It also promotes the growth of beneficial gut bacteria, which play a crucial role in digestion, nutrient absorption, and overall gut health.

6. Mental Health: Proper nutrition is closely linked to mental well-being. A balanced diet that includes essential nutrients like omega-3 fatty acids, B vitamins, and antioxidants can support brain health, mood regulation, and cognitive function. On the other hand, a poor

diet lacking in essential nutrients may contribute to mental health issues such as depression and anxiety.

Remember, a balanced diet is not about strict rules or deprivation but rather about making healthy choices and finding a sustainable approach to nourishing your body. Consulting a registered dietitian or nutritionist can help you create a personalized and balanced eating plan based on your individual needs and goals.

B. Nutritional considerations for individuals over 40

As we age, our nutritional needs and considerations may change. Here are some key nutritional considerations for individuals over 40:

1. Nutrient-Dense Foods: As we age, our metabolism slows down, and our bodies may require fewer calories. It becomes even more important to focus on nutrient-dense foods that provide essential vitamins, minerals, and other beneficial compounds. Include plenty of fruits, vegetables, whole grains, lean proteins, and healthy fats in your diet.

2. Calcium and Vitamin D: The risk of osteoporosis increases with age, especially for women. Adequate calcium and vitamin D intake are essential for maintaining bone health. Include dairy products, leafy greens, fortified foods, and supplements if necessary to meet your calcium and vitamin D needs.

3. Fiber: Age-related changes in the digestive system can lead to constipation. Consuming adequate fiber helps maintain regular bowel movements and supports digestive health. Include whole grains, fruits, vegetables, legumes, and nuts in your diet to increase your fiber intake.

4. Hydration: Staying well-hydrated is important for individuals of all ages. As we age, the sense of thirst may diminish, making it easier to become dehydrated. Ensure you drink enough water throughout the day, and include hydrating foods such as fruits and vegetables in your diet.

5. Omega-3 Fatty Acids: Omega-3 fatty acids have been shown to have numerous health benefits, including reducing the risk of heart disease and inflammation. Include fatty fish (such as salmon and sardines), flaxseeds, chia seeds, and walnuts in your diet to increase your omega-3 fatty acid intake.

6. Protein: Protein is important for maintaining muscle mass, which tends to decline with age. Aim to include lean sources of protein such as poultry, fish, legumes, tofu, and dairy products in your meals. Distribute your protein intake evenly throughout the day to support muscle synthesis.

7. Antioxidants: Antioxidants help protect the body from cellular damage caused by free radicals. Include a variety of colorful fruits and vegetables in your diet to increase your antioxidant intake. Berries, dark leafy greens, citrus fruits, and cruciferous vegetables are particularly rich in antioxidants.

8. Regular Physical Activity: Along with proper nutrition, regular physical activity is crucial for maintaining overall health. Engage in a combination of aerobic exercise, strength training, and flexibility exercises to support your physical and mental well-being as you age.

Remember, these considerations are general guidelines, and individual needs may vary. It is always a good idea to consult with a healthcare professional or registered dietitian to create a personalized nutrition plan based on your specific needs, medical history, and goals.

C. Staying hydrated and the role of water in maintaining vitality

Staying hydrated is essential for maintaining vitality and overall well-being. Water plays several important roles in our bodies:

1. Optimal Body Function: Water is involved in numerous bodily functions, including digestion, absorption, circulation, and temperature regulation. It helps transport nutrients, remove waste, lubricate joints, and support organ function.

2. Energy Levels: Dehydration can lead to fatigue and decreased energy levels. When we don't drink enough water, our bodies may struggle to carry out basic functions efficiently, leaving us feeling tired and sluggish. Staying hydrated can help maintain energy and improve focus.

3. Brain Function: Our brains are highly dependent on adequate hydration to function optimally. Even mild dehydration can affect cognitive performance, mood, and memory. Drinking enough water can help improve concentration and mental clarity.

4. Physical Performance: During exercise or physical activity, our bodies lose water through sweat. Dehydration can negatively impact performance, leading to decreased endurance, reduced strength, and increased fatigue. Proper hydration before, during, and after physical activity is crucial for optimal performance and recovery.

5. Digestive Health: Water plays a vital role in digestion and preventing constipation. It helps break down food, aids in nutrient absorption, and facilitates smooth bowel movements. Insufficient water intake can lead to digestive issues and discomfort.

Tips for staying hydrated and maintaining vitality:

1. Drink Enough Water: Aim to drink at least 8 cups (64 ounces) of water per day, or more if you're physically active or live in a hot climate. Carry a reusable water bottle with you to remind yourself to drink throughout the day.

2. Monitor Urine Color: Pay attention to the color of your urine. If it's light yellow or clear, it indicates that you're properly hydrated. Dark yellow urine may be a sign of dehydration, so increase your water intake.

3. Hydrating Foods: Include hydrating foods in your diet, such as fruits (watermelon, oranges, strawberries), vegetables (cucumbers, lettuce, celery), and soups. These foods contain high water content and can contribute to your overall hydration.

4. Limit Caffeine and Alcohol: Both caffeine and alcohol can have diuretic effects, increasing fluid loss and potentially contributing to dehydration. If you consume these beverages, balance them with additional water intake.

5. Listen to Your Body: Thirst is a reliable indicator that your body needs water. Drink when you feel thirsty, and don't wait until you're extremely thirsty.

Remember, individual hydration needs may vary based on factors such as activity level, climate, and health conditions. It's always beneficial to consult with a healthcare professional for personalized recommendations.

VIII. Rest and Recovery

A. Recognizing the importance of rest for optimal performance

Rest is indeed crucial for optimal performance. Here are some key points highlighting the importance of rest:

1. Physical Recovery: Rest allows our bodies to repair and regenerate. It helps muscles recover from exercise, reduces the risk of injury, and improves overall physical performance.

2. Mental Rejuvenation: Resting helps clear our minds, reduce stress, and improve mental well-being. It enhances focus, concentration, and cognitive function, leading to better performance in various tasks.

3. Improved Productivity: Taking regular breaks and getting sufficient sleep can actually enhance productivity. It prevents burnout, improves decision-making abilities, and allows for better creativity and problem-solving skills.

4. Enhanced Learning and Memory: Rest plays a vital role in memory consolidation and learning. Quality sleep and downtime enable our brains to process and retain information effectively, leading to improved learning outcomes.

5. Energy Restoration: Rest replenishes our energy levels. It allows us to recharge both physically and mentally, leading to increased stamina, endurance, and overall performance in daily activities.

6. Mental and Emotional Balance: Rest helps maintain a healthy balance in our mental and emotional states. It reduces the risk of mood disorders, improves emotional resilience, and promotes overall well-being.

Remember, finding the right balance between activity and rest is essential for optimal performance. It's important to prioritize self-care and incorporate restful practices into our daily routines to achieve long-term success and well-being.

B. Prioritizing quality sleep and relaxation techniques

Prioritizing quality sleep and incorporating relaxation techniques into your routine can greatly benefit your overall well-being and performance. Here are some tips:

1. Establish a Consistent Sleep Schedule: Try to go to bed and wake up at the same time every day, even on weekends. This helps regulate your body's internal clock and promotes better sleep quality.

2. Create a Sleep-Friendly Environment: Make your bedroom a comfortable and relaxing space. Keep the room cool, dark, and quiet. Consider using earplugs, eye masks, or white noise machines if needed.

3. Limit Exposure to Electronic Devices: The blue light emitted by electronic devices can disrupt your sleep. Avoid using smartphones, tablets, or computers for at least an hour before bedtime. Instead, engage in calming activities like reading a book or practicing relaxation techniques.

4. Practice Relaxation Techniques: Incorporate relaxation techniques into your daily routine. This could include deep breathing exercises, meditation, progressive muscle relaxation, or guided imagery. These techniques help reduce stress, calm the mind, and prepare your body for restful sleep.

5. Create a Bedtime Routine: Establish a relaxing routine before bed to signal to your body that it's time to wind down. This could involve taking a warm bath, listening to soothing music, or practicing gentle stretching or yoga.

6. Limit Stimulants: Avoid consuming caffeine, nicotine, and alcohol close to bedtime, as they can disrupt your sleep patterns. Opt for herbal teas or decaffeinated beverages instead.

7. Avoid Heavy Meals and Exercise Before Bed: Eating a heavy meal or engaging in intense exercise close to bedtime can interfere with sleep. Try to eat your last meal at least a few hours before bed and finish any vigorous exercise earlier in the day.

8. Create a Comfortable Sleep Environment: Invest in a supportive mattress and comfortable pillows that suit your preferences. Choose breathable and lightweight bedding to help regulate body temperature during sleep.

Remember, everyone's sleep needs are different. Pay attention to your body's signals and adjust your sleep routine accordingly. Prioritizing quality sleep and incorporating relaxation techniques can have a significant positive impact on your overall performance, health, and well-being.

C. Listening to the body and allowing time for recovery

Listening to the cues of your body and providing ample time for recovery are of utmost importance when it comes to maintaining optimal health and performance. Let us delve deeper into this topic, exploring key aspects that warrant our attention:

1. Attuning to Physical Indicators: Your body possesses an innate ability to communicate its needs, often manifesting through signals such as sensations of weariness, muscle tenderness, or a decline in performance. Honoring and heeding these signals is crucial, as pushing yourself beyond your limits without affording your body the necessary recovery time can result in burnout and an increased susceptibility to injuries.

2. Embracing Restorative Sleep: Prioritizing high-quality sleep is paramount in facilitating recovery. Striving to attain a consistent duration of 7-9 hours of uninterrupted sleep each night allows your body to initiate its repair processes and replenish its energy reserves.

3. Incorporating Rest Days: Integrating regular rest days into your exercise regimen is vital for optimizing recovery. These designated periods of respite enable your muscles, joints, and nervous system to recuperate from the stresses incurred during training. Utilize these days to engage in gentle activities, such as stretching, yoga, or leisurely walks, as they promote blood circulation and aid in the recovery process.

4. Active Recovery: In addition to traditional rest days, consider integrating active recovery exercises into your routine. These low-impact activities, including swimming, cycling, or light stretching, stimulate blood flow to the muscles, help eliminate metabolic waste, and facilitate the healing process.

5. Attentiveness to Pain and Discomfort: It is crucial to attentively listen to your body when it communicates pain or discomfort during or after physical exertion. Ignoring these signals can exacerbate injuries and prolong the recovery timeline. If necessary, seek guidance from healthcare professionals to ensure appropriate treatment and rehabilitation.

6. Nourishing Nutrition: Fueling your body with a well-balanced, nutrient-dense diet is fundamental for optimal recovery. Concentrate on consuming lean proteins, healthy fats, fruits, vegetables, and whole grains, as these elements support muscle repair, mitigate inflammation, and provide the energy required for the recovery process.

7. Hydration: Maintaining proper hydration throughout the day is paramount, as water plays a vital role in numerous bodily functions, including recovery. Strive to drink an adequate amount of water to maintain clear urine and replenish fluids lost during physical activity.

8. Stress Management: Chronic stress can impede the body's ability to recover effectively. Integrating stress management techniques, such as mindfulness, meditation, or engaging in pleasurable hobbies, fosters relaxation and diminishes stress levels, thus promoting the recovery process.

It is essential to recognize that recovery is a highly individualized journey, necessitating an attentive ear to your body's unique needs. By allowing ample time for recovery and attentively heeding your body's cues, you can enhance your overall well-being and optimize your performance levels.

IX. Mind-Body Connection

A. Incorporating mindfulness and stress management techniques

Incorporating mindfulness and stress management techniques can greatly contribute to maintaining vitality and overall well-being. Here are some strategies to help you cultivate mindfulness and manage stress:

1. Deep Breathing: Take slow, deep breaths in through your nose and exhale through your mouth. Focusing on your breath can help calm your mind and relax your body. Practice deep breathing exercises whenever you feel stressed or overwhelmed.

2. Meditation: Set aside a few minutes each day for meditation. Find a quiet and comfortable space, close your eyes, and focus your attention on your breath, a specific sensation, or a guided meditation. Meditation can help reduce stress, improve focus, and promote a sense of inner calm.

3. Mindful Eating: Pay attention to the experience of eating. Slow down, savor each bite, and fully engage your senses. Notice the flavors, textures, and smells of your food. Mindful eating can help prevent overeating, enhance digestion, and promote a healthier relationship with food.

4. Nature Walks: Take regular walks outdoors and immerse yourself in nature. Pay attention to the sights, sounds, and sensations around you. Engaging with nature can help reduce stress, boost mood, and increase feelings of well-being.

5. Journaling: Write down your thoughts, feelings, and experiences in a journal. This practice can help you gain clarity, process emotions, and release stress. Set aside a few minutes each day to reflect on your day or engage in gratitude journaling, where you write down things you're grateful for.

6. Mindful Movement: Engage in activities that promote mindful movement, such as yoga, tai chi, or qigong. These practices combine physical movement with breath awareness, helping to reduce stress, improve flexibility, and enhance mind-body connection.

7. Digital Detox: Take regular breaks from technology and screens. Disconnecting from constant digital stimulation can help reduce stress and promote a greater sense of presence and mindfulness in your daily life.

8. Prioritize Self-Care: Engage in activities that nourish your body and mind. This can include getting enough sleep, eating nutritious meals, engaging in hobbies, spending time with loved ones, and practicing relaxation techniques.

Remember, incorporating mindfulness and stress management techniques is a personal journey. Find what works best for you and be consistent in your practice. If you feel overwhelmed, don't hesitate to seek support from a mental health professional or join a mindfulness-based program.

B. Benefits of meditation, deep breathing, and visualization

Meditation, deep breathing, and visualization are powerful practices that offer a wide range of benefits. Here are some of the key benefits of each:

1. Meditation:

- Reduces stress and anxiety: Regular meditation practice can help to calm the mind and alleviate stress, promoting a greater sense of inner peace and relaxation.
- Improves focus and concentration: By training the mind to stay present and focused, meditation can enhance cognitive function and improve productivity.
- Boosts emotional well-being: Meditation cultivates mindfulness and self-awareness, allowing you to better understand and regulate your emotions.
- Enhances overall mental health: Research suggests that meditation can help reduce symptoms of depression, improve sleep quality, and increase overall psychological well-being.

2. Deep Breathing:
- Relaxes the body and mind: Deep breathing triggers the release of endorphins, promoting relaxation and reducing tension in the body.
- Lowers blood pressure and heart rate: By activating the body's relaxation response, deep breathing can help to reduce blood pressure and heart rate, promoting cardiovascular health.
- Improves respiratory function: Deep breathing exercises can strengthen the respiratory muscles and increase lung capacity, leading to improved oxygen intake and better overall lung function.
- Enhances mental clarity: Deep breathing techniques provide a quick and effective way to clear the mind, increase focus, and reduce mental fatigue.

3. Visualization:
- Increases motivation and goal attainment: Visualizing your goals and desired outcomes can enhance motivation and increase the likelihood of achieving them.
- Reduces stress and anxiety: Visualization can create a sense of calm and relaxation, reducing stress and anxiety levels.
- Enhances performance: Athletes and performers often use visualization techniques to improve their skills and enhance performance by mentally rehearsing successful outcomes.
- Boosts self-confidence: By visualizing positive scenarios and outcomes, you can cultivate a greater sense of self-belief and confidence.

Overall, incorporating meditation, deep breathing, and visualization into your daily routine can have a positive impact on your physical, mental, and emotional well-being, helping you lead a more balanced and fulfilling life.

C. Practicing self-care and nurturing the mind-body connection

Practicing self-care and nurturing the mind-body connection is essential for overall well-being. Here are some ways you can cultivate self-care and strengthen the mind-body connection:

1. Prioritize self-care activities: Set aside dedicated time each day or week for activities that nourish your mind, body, and soul. This can include things like taking a bath, reading a book, going for a walk in nature, practicing yoga, or engaging in a hobby that brings you joy.

2. Practice mindfulness: Mindfulness involves paying attention to the present moment without judgment. Engaging in mindfulness exercises, such as meditation or mindful breathing, can help you become more aware of your thoughts, emotions, and physical sensations. This awareness can lead to better self-care choices and a stronger mind-body connection.

3. Engage in regular exercise: Physical activity not only benefits your body but also has a positive impact on your mental well-being. Engaging in regular exercise releases endorphins, reduces stress, improves mood, and enhances cognitive function. Find activities that you enjoy, whether it's jogging, dancing, swimming, or practicing yoga, and make it a part of your self-care routine.

4. Get enough restful sleep: Sleep is crucial for both your physical and mental health. Prioritize getting enough sleep by establishing a regular sleep schedule, creating a calming bedtime routine, and creating a sleep-conducive environment. Quality sleep rejuvenates your body and mind, allowing you to better handle daily challenges and nurture the mind-body connection.

5. Practice healthy eating habits: Nourishing your body with a balanced diet can have a significant impact on your overall well-

being. Focus on consuming whole, nutrient-dense foods that fuel your body and support brain health. Stay hydrated, limit processed foods, and listen to your body's hunger and fullness cues.

6. Connect with supportive relationships: Foster relationships with people who uplift and support you. Social connections play a crucial role in self-care and nurturing the mind-body connection. Surrounding yourself with positive and supportive individuals can boost your mood, reduce stress, and provide a sense of belonging.

Remember, self-care is a personal journey, and it's important to find what works best for you. By prioritizing self-care activities and nurturing the mind-body connection, you can enhance your overall well-being and lead a more fulfilling life.

X. Social Connections and Mental Stimulation

A. Importance of social interactions for mental well-being

Social interactions play a vital role in maintaining and promoting mental well-being. Here are some reasons why social interactions are important:

1. Emotional support: Engaging in social interactions allows us to connect with others and receive emotional support. Sharing our thoughts, feelings, and experiences with trusted individuals can help us process emotions, alleviate stress, and gain new perspectives. Having a support system can make us feel understood, valued, and less alone, which can have a positive impact on our mental well-being.

2. Reduced feelings of loneliness: Loneliness can have detrimental effects on mental health. Regular social interactions help combat feelings of isolation and loneliness. Being part of a community, whether it's a close-knit group of friends, family, or a larger social network, provides a sense of belonging and can improve overall mental well-being.

3. Enhanced self-esteem: Social interactions can boost self-esteem and self-worth. When we engage with others in positive and meaningful ways, we receive validation and recognition, which can positively impact our self-perception. Surrounding ourselves with supportive individuals who appreciate and respect us can help us build a healthy self-image and maintain a positive mindset.

4. Stress reduction: Spending time with others and engaging in social activities can help reduce stress levels. Social interactions provide opportunities for laughter, relaxation, and enjoyable experiences, which can alleviate stress and improve our mood. Additionally, sharing our concerns and challenges with trusted individuals can provide different perspectives and coping strategies, helping us navigate stressful situations more effectively.

5. Cognitive stimulation: Social interactions stimulate our minds and promote cognitive health. Engaging in conversations, debates, or even playing games with others challenges our thinking, expands our knowledge, and keeps our minds active. This cognitive stimulation can contribute to improved mental well-being and overall brain health.

6. Increased resilience: Social interactions can enhance our resilience and ability to cope with life's challenges. Having a support system can provide a sense of stability and security during difficult times. Through social interactions, we can share experiences, seek advice, and gain encouragement, which can help us navigate adversity and bounce back from setbacks.

In summary, social interactions are crucial for mental well-being. They provide emotional support, reduce loneliness, boost self-esteem, help manage stress, stimulate cognition, and enhance resilience. Prioritizing and nurturing social connections can significantly contribute to our overall mental health and happiness.

B. Engaging in intellectual and creative pursuits

Engaging in intellectual and creative pursuits is not only enjoyable but also beneficial for our mental well-being. Here are some reasons why these activities are important:

1. Cognitive stimulation: Intellectual and creative pursuits challenge our minds and help keep our brains active. They involve problem-solving, critical thinking, and creativity, which can improve cognitive function and enhance mental agility. Regularly engaging in such activities can help sharpen our focus, expand our knowledge, and improve overall cognitive abilities.

2. Stress reduction: Immersing ourselves in intellectual and creative pursuits can be a great way to unwind and relax. These activities provide an outlet for self-expression, allowing us to channel our thoughts and emotions in a positive and productive manner. They can act as a form of therapy, helping us manage stress, reduce anxiety, and promote a sense of calm and well-being.

3. Personal growth: Intellectual and creative pursuits provide opportunities for personal growth and self-discovery. They allow us to explore new interests, talents, and passions. Engaging in these activities can help us develop new skills, expand our horizons, and gain a deeper understanding of ourselves and the world around us. This sense of personal growth can contribute to increased self-confidence and a greater sense of fulfillment.

4. Social connections: Intellectual and creative pursuits often involve connecting with others who share similar interests. Whether it's joining a book club, participating in a painting class, or engaging in intellectual discussions, these activities can provide opportunities to meet like-minded individuals and build meaningful social connections. Connecting with others who share our passions can lead to a sense of belonging and foster a supportive community.

5. Increased happiness and well-being: Engaging in intellectual and creative pursuits can bring a sense of joy, fulfillment, and satisfaction. These activities allow us to tap into our creativity, express ourselves, and pursue our passions. When we engage in

activities that align with our interests and values, it can contribute to a greater sense of purpose and overall happiness in life.

6. Improved problem-solving skills: Intellectual and creative pursuits often require us to think outside the box and come up with innovative solutions. By regularly challenging ourselves in these activities, we can enhance our problem-solving skills, adaptability, and creativity. These skills can be valuable in various aspects of life, from personal relationships to professional endeavors.

In summary, engaging in intellectual and creative pursuits offers numerous benefits for our mental well-being. They stimulate our minds, reduce stress, foster personal growth, facilitate social connections, increase happiness, and improve problem-solving skills. So, whether it's reading, writing, painting, playing an instrument, or engaging in intellectual discussions, incorporating these pursuits into our lives can have a positive impact on our overall mental health and satisfaction.

C. Seeking new experiences and staying socially active

Seeking new experiences and staying socially active are important aspects of personal growth and well-being. Here's why:

1. Personal growth: Seeking new experiences allows us to step out of our comfort zones and expand our horizons. It exposes us to different perspectives, cultures, and ideas, which can broaden our understanding of the world and ourselves. Trying new things challenges us to learn, adapt, and grow, leading to personal development and a greater sense of self-confidence.

2. Learning and knowledge: Engaging in new experiences provides opportunities for learning and acquiring new skills. Whether it's taking up a new hobby, exploring a new place, or trying a new activity, each experience offers something to learn. These experiences can stimulate our curiosity, enhance our knowledge, and keep our minds active and engaged.

3. Breaking routine: Routine can sometimes lead to monotony and boredom. Seeking new experiences helps break the cycle and adds

excitement and variety to our lives. It injects a sense of novelty and adventure, making each day more interesting and fulfilling. Breaking routine can also boost creativity and inspire us to think in new and innovative ways.

4. Social connections: Staying socially active is crucial for maintaining meaningful relationships and a strong support network. Engaging with others through social activities, clubs, volunteering, or joining interest groups allows us to meet new people, make friends, and foster a sense of belonging. Social connections contribute to our overall happiness, well-being, and provide a support system during both challenging and joyful times.

5. Emotional well-being: Seeking new experiences and staying socially active can positively impact our emotional well-being. It provides opportunities for social interaction, laughter, and shared experiences, which can boost mood, reduce feelings of loneliness, and enhance overall happiness. Engaging in activities that bring us joy and fulfillment can also serve as a form of self-care, improving our mental and emotional health.

6. Adaptability and resilience: Seeking new experiences helps develop adaptability and resilience. It exposes us to unfamiliar situations and challenges, requiring us to navigate through them and adapt to new environments. These experiences can help us become more flexible, open-minded, and better equipped to handle change and uncertainty in life.

In summary, seeking new experiences and staying socially active contribute to personal growth, learning, breaking routine, building social connections, enhancing emotional well-being, and developing adaptability. By embracing new opportunities and engaging with others, we can lead more fulfilling lives, continuously learn and grow, and create lasting memories and relationships.

XI. Regular Health Check-Ups

A. Monitoring overall health and well-being

Monitoring overall health and well-being is crucial for maintaining a happy and healthy lifestyle. Here are some key points to consider:

1. Regular check-ups: Scheduling routine check-ups with healthcare professionals, such as doctors and dentists, is essential for monitoring your overall health. These check-ups can help identify any potential health issues early on and allow for timely intervention and treatment.

2. Physical activity: Engaging in regular physical activity is vital for maintaining good physical and mental health. It helps improve cardiovascular health, strengthens muscles and bones, and reduces the risk of chronic diseases. Tracking your physical activity levels, whether through wearable devices or simply keeping a log, can help you stay motivated and ensure you're meeting your fitness goals.

3. Balanced diet: A well-balanced diet plays a significant role in maintaining overall health. Monitoring your nutritional intake, such as tracking your macronutrients (carbohydrates, proteins, and fats) and micronutrients (vitamins and minerals), can help ensure you're getting the necessary nutrients your body needs. Consulting with a registered dietitian can provide personalized guidance based on your specific dietary needs.

4. Sleep patterns: Quality sleep is essential for physical and mental restoration. Monitoring your sleep patterns, including duration and quality, can help identify any sleep disturbances or issues. Maintaining a consistent sleep routine, creating a sleep-friendly environment, and practicing good sleep hygiene can contribute to better sleep and overall well-being.

5. Mental well-being: Paying attention to your mental health is equally important. Monitoring your emotional well-being, stress levels, and mood can help identify any signs of anxiety, depression, or other mental health concerns. Engaging in activities that promote relaxation and self-care, such as meditation, mindfulness, or hobbies you enjoy, can contribute to better mental and emotional well-being.

6. Social support: Maintaining strong social connections is crucial for overall well-being. Regularly checking in with friends, family, or participating in social activities can provide emotional support and reduce feelings of loneliness. Social support is essential for managing stress, boosting happiness, and maintaining a sense of belonging.

7. Stress management: Chronic stress can negatively impact your health and well-being. Monitoring your stress levels and identifying stressors can help you develop effective strategies to manage stress. Engaging in stress-reducing activities, such as exercise, relaxation techniques, or seeking professional help, can contribute to better overall health.

In summary, monitoring overall health and well-being involves regular check-ups, tracking physical activity and nutrition, paying attention to sleep patterns and mental well-being, maintaining social connections, and managing stress effectively. By being proactive and mindful of these aspects, you can take control of your health and well-being, leading to a healthier and more fulfilling life.

B. Importance of regular medical check-ups and screenings

Regular medical check-ups and screenings are vital for maintaining good health and preventing potential health issues. Here are some reasons why they are important:

1. Early detection of diseases: Regular check-ups allow healthcare professionals to assess your overall health and identify any signs or symptoms of potential diseases or conditions at an early stage. Early detection often leads to more effective treatment and better health outcomes.

2. Prevention and health promotion: Check-ups provide an opportunity for preventive care, including vaccinations, screenings, and counseling on healthy lifestyle habits. Through screenings, healthcare professionals can identify risk factors and provide guidance on how to reduce those risks and improve your overall well-being.

3. Monitoring chronic conditions: If you have a chronic condition, regular check-ups are crucial for monitoring its progression and managing it effectively. Healthcare professionals can adjust treatment plans, medications, or lifestyle recommendations based on your evolving health needs.

4. Health education and guidance: Check-ups offer an opportunity for healthcare professionals to educate and provide guidance on various health topics. They can address your questions, provide information on healthy habits, and offer personalized advice tailored to your specific health needs.

5. Mental health assessment: Regular check-ups also encompass mental health assessments, as mental well-being is an essential aspect of overall health. Healthcare professionals can evaluate your mental health status, provide support, and refer you to specialists if necessary.

6. Building a trusted relationship with healthcare providers: Regular check-ups help establish a strong relationship with your healthcare provider. This relationship fosters open communication, trust, and collaboration, allowing for better healthcare decision-making and personalized care.

7. Monitoring overall health trends: By having regular check-ups and screenings, your healthcare provider can monitor your health over time and track any changes or trends. This information can help identify patterns, make informed decisions, and catch any potential health issues before they become more serious.

In summary, regular medical check-ups and screenings are essential for early detection, prevention, disease management, health education, mental health assessment, and establishing a trusted relationship with healthcare providers. By prioritizing these check-ups, you can take a proactive approach to your health, leading to better overall well-being and potentially avoiding more serious health complications in the future.

C. Addressing any concerns or changes in physical condition

Addressing concerns or changes in your physical condition is an important aspect of maintaining good health. If you notice any unusual symptoms or changes in your body, it is recommended to take the following steps:

1. Document your symptoms: Make a note of any specific symptoms you are experiencing, including when they started, their frequency, and any factors that may worsen or alleviate them. This information will be helpful when discussing your concerns with a healthcare professional.

2. Consult with a healthcare professional: Schedule an appointment with your primary care physician or an appropriate specialist to discuss your concerns. Explain your symptoms, any changes you have observed, and any relevant medical history. They can evaluate your condition, ask further questions, and perform any necessary examinations or tests.

3. Be open and honest: During your appointment, be open and honest with your healthcare professional. Provide them with accurate information about your symptoms, lifestyle habits, medications, and any other relevant details. This will help them make an accurate diagnosis and develop an appropriate treatment plan.

4. Ask questions: Don't hesitate to ask questions about your concerns or any changes you're experiencing. Seek clarification on any medical terms or recommendations that you don't understand. Understanding your condition and treatment options will empower you to make informed decisions about your health.

5. Follow the recommended treatment plan: If your healthcare professional diagnoses a condition or recommends a treatment plan, it is important to follow their advice. This may include lifestyle modifications, medications, therapy, or other interventions. Adhering to the recommended plan can improve your condition and overall well-being.

6. Seek a second opinion if necessary: If you are unsure about a diagnosis or treatment plan, or if you do not feel satisfied with the

care you are receiving, it is entirely appropriate to seek a second opinion from another healthcare professional. It's important to feel comfortable and confident in your medical care.

Remember, addressing concerns or changes in your physical condition promptly can help prevent potential complications and lead to better health outcomes. By seeking appropriate medical attention and actively participating in your healthcare, you are taking an important step towards maintaining your well-being.

XII. Conclusion

A. Recap of key points and takeaways

Here's a recap of the key points and takeaways for addressing concerns or changes in your physical condition:

1. Document your symptoms: Keep track of specific symptoms, their frequency, and any factors that may affect them.

2. Consult with a healthcare professional: Schedule an appointment with your primary care physician or a specialist to discuss your concerns.

3. Be open and honest: Provide accurate information about your symptoms, lifestyle habits, medications, and medical history.

4. Ask questions: Seek clarification and ask questions about your concerns, diagnosis, and treatment options.

5. Follow the recommended treatment plan: Adhere to the advice and treatment plan provided by your healthcare professional.

6. Seek a second opinion if necessary: If you're unsure or unsatisfied, don't hesitate to seek a second opinion.

By following these steps, you can ensure that your concerns are addressed promptly and accurately, leading to better health outcomes. Remember, your health is important, and seeking appropriate medical attention is crucial for maintaining your well-being.

B. Encouragement to embrace an active and youthful lifestyle

Embracing an active and youthful lifestyle can have numerous benefits for your physical and mental well-being. Here are some encouraging points to help you get started:

1. Increased energy levels: Regular physical activity can boost your energy levels and combat feelings of fatigue. You'll feel more active and productive throughout the day.

2. Improved physical health: Engaging in exercise and maintaining an active lifestyle can help prevent chronic diseases like heart disease, diabetes, and certain cancers. It also strengthens your immune system.

3. Enhances mental well-being: Exercise releases endorphins, which are natural mood boosters. It can reduce stress, anxiety, and symptoms of depression, promoting a positive mindset.

4. Maintains a healthy weight: Regular physical activity, along with a balanced diet, can help you maintain a healthy weight and body composition.

5. Increased mobility and flexibility: Staying active helps improve joint flexibility, muscle strength, and overall mobility. This can enhance your independence and quality of life as you age.

6. Social engagement: Participating in activities like group sports or fitness classes offers opportunities to meet new people, build friendships, and create a supportive social network.

Remember, it's never too late to start. Start small, gradually increase your activity level, and find activities you enjoy. Whether it's walking, dancing, swimming, or any other form of exercise, find what brings you joy and make it a regular part of your routine. Embracing an active and youthful lifestyle can lead to a happier, healthier, and more fulfilling life.

C. Empowering individuals over 40 to say "FU" to getting old and live their best lives

Absolutely! It's time to say "FU" to getting old and live your best life, regardless of age. Here's how you can empower yourself and embrace a vibrant and fulfilling life:

1. Embrace a positive mindset: Age is just a number, and it doesn't define your worth or capabilities. Believe in yourself and focus on the positive aspects of aging, like wisdom, experience, and the opportunity for personal growth.

2. Prioritize self-care: Take care of your physical, mental, and emotional well-being. Make time for activities that bring you joy and relaxation, whether it's practicing mindfulness, indulging in hobbies, or pampering yourself.

3. Stay active and embrace fitness: Engage in regular physical activity that suits your abilities and preferences. Whether it's yoga, weightlifting, dancing, or any other form of exercise, find what keeps you motivated and energized. Remember, it's never too late to start and reap the benefits of an active lifestyle.

4. Nourish your body: Focus on a well-balanced diet that includes plenty of fruits, vegetables, lean proteins, and whole grains. Stay hydrated, limit processed foods, and indulge in moderation. Taking care of your body from the inside will help you feel and look your best.

5. Challenge yourself: Don't be afraid to step out of your comfort zone and try new things. Take up new hobbies, learn new skills, or pursue goals and dreams you've always had. Embracing new challenges keeps your mind sharp and stimulates personal growth.

6. Cultivate meaningful relationships: Surround yourself with positive and supportive people who uplift and inspire you. Build strong connections with family, friends, and like-minded individuals who share your passion for living life to the fullest.

Remember, age is just a number, and you have the power to create a life that's fulfilling, vibrant, and full of joy. Say "FU" to getting old and embrace each day with enthusiasm and determination to live your best life.

Dear readers,

Thank you so much for taking the time to read the book! I truly appreciate your support and interest in empowering individuals over 40 to live their best lives. Your feedback and thoughts on the book are incredibly valuable.

If you enjoyed the book and found it helpful, I would kindly ask you to consider leaving an honest review. Your review can help others discover the book and decide if it's the right fit for them. Whether it's on a retailer's website, a book review platform, or even sharing your thoughts with friends and family, your review can make a significant impact.

I'm grateful for your support and would love to hear your thoughts. Reviews not only help me as an author but also contribute to building a supportive community of individuals who are embracing life and saying "FU" to getting old. Thank you again, and I look forward to hearing your feedback!

www.ingramcontent.com/pod-product-compliance
Lightning Source LLC
Chambersburg PA
CBHW071005260726
48661CB00007B/2796